Practical Management for Charge Nurses

By Harry G. Baum, Ed. D.

Practical Management for Charge Nurses

By Harry G. Baum, Ed. D.

Copyright ©2011 Harry G. Baum, Ed. D.

Published by MeritCare Health Systems, Inc.

For additional information, please contact the author at:

harry_g_baum@msn.com

Cover illustration by:

Brigitte St-Pierre

Printed in the United States

Practical Management for Charge Nurses

ISBN 10: 098345020X

ISBN 13: 978-0983450207

The interface between one's direct supervisor and the staff member providing fundamental aspects of the job is never so important than when working within a human service profession and even more significant when working in healthcare. It is difficult to go back and fix a mistake, catch and issue that should have been caught sooner, or rebuild relationships of trust with patients and family members. Dr. Baum's understanding of managerial leadership cuts straight to the essence of the challenge of providing line staff with vision and motivation while at the same time giving them the direction and accountability they need to stay on task.

Many healthcare facilities suffer from a systems flow issue where the information and workload flowing from one shift to the next is inconsistent and misdirected. Dr. Baum focus on this issue presents a practical guide to nurses. The information provided has a potential to yield great benefits to any organization wishing to improve the quality of their services and reduce the confusion that so often results in customer dissatisfaction and staff turnover. Because of the human element, healthcare professionals are constantly working to balance a busy load with a dynamic environment. Keeping staff motivated throughout the workday and being on top of the many changing issues is paramount to success.

This book lights the way for supervisors to communicate in a manner that provides staff they are directly supervising with the insight, expectations, incentive and accountability to provide effective, efficient quality care to patients, family members and to one another. Principles delineated in this document are fundamental to the success of each healthcare professional regardless of the environment or position. Enjoy the read, but most importantly, apply the principles.

~ Fred Hermes, Owner/CEO, Axiom Healthcare Management

Table of Contents

Acknowledgements

I would like to dedicate this book to my family – my wife Connie, my daughters Kirstin, Angela, and Jennifer, and my son Brian. I would also like to thank them and their families for all the support they have given to our business throughout the years. They will one day have the honor of owning our business and caring for the great people for whom we care, and I know they will continue to make us proud.

Preface

It has been my experience in post-acute and long-term care that charge nurses have an extremely difficult and often demanding job to do. Their school experience only partially prepares them for the rigors of the actual work world. Most schools prepare a nurse for 75% of the technical skills they need to take care of patients, but do not provide any practical skills of preparation for organizing and managing a job.

Charge nurses are expected to go directly from school, do not pass "GO", go directly to what feels like "jail" to them, and then miraculously be all things to all people in a new job. This book offers some practical insights into what I think will help a charge nurse manage her position, and, in turn, be able to take better care of the residents for whom she is responsible.

My hope is that the new nurse or even the experienced nurse who is having difficulty handling the stress of the job will read and refer to the chapters in this book and carry it with her until she becomes comfortable in the concepts presented. I attempted to put practical examples in the book to allow the nurse to apply them to everyday situations.

I hope it helps charge nurses become more confident and much more prepared when taking care of the individuals that deserve it the most: themselves and their patients.

(Dr. Harry Baum)

History of Sharon Lane

Fostering a sense of community within a community, Sharon Lane Health Services provides the foundation of family. At Sharon Lane, our residents are treated like members of our own family, and our highly skilled and dedicated staff of team players strives to offer our residents the same spirit of independence they have come to appreciate their whole lives. We provide a positive and stimulating skilled nursing environment with complete attention on the physical, emotional, and spiritual care of each resident, affording them their dignity and sense of purpose. At Sharon Lane, we believe going home means coming home.

Sharon Lane Health Services believes in the team approach in its efforts to provide a caring environment for our residents. In fact, each of our three established care units is organized into a specific team.

The concept behind the team approach is to provide enhanced care for our residents by not only getting to know them, but through developing relationships with their families and by striving to understand and appreciate their histories and life stories. These are individuals, each with a unique story and personality. Through our appreciation and understanding of those, we get to know them better and can greatly improve on our ability to serve them through our daily tasks.

Each team consists of all the individuals from every department that work with the residents on that unit.

The unit is organized with a group of team leaders. These leaders are responsible for developing team goals, motivating team members, communicating information to the team, listening to concerns of the team, solving problems for the team, being spokespersons for the team, and evaluating the team's progress toward goals.

Sharon Lane Health Services believes that this approach provides a sense of home and a comforting, familiar environment for our residents. We believe that this approach will give our residents the opportunity to be "The Best That They Can Be!"

That sense of welcoming comfort is also extended to the families of our residents. Our competent staff assists them through the financial process, both in the understanding of and the implementation of such matters. We accept private pay, HMO, Medicare, Medicaid, long-term care insurance and Veteran's Administration residents'.

Contrary to the old way of care-giving, Sharon Lane regards its resident's satisfaction first, with the understanding that true happiness lies in self-determination. That is why the caregiver and homemaker staff will make every effort to get to know residents on a personal level, referred to as consistent staffing. This provides residents with the tools needed to make sound, healthy decisions on their own behalf.

Ultimately, by placing the resident's ability to make his or her own choices concerning care and daily living as a higher priority than simple operational efficiency or staff convenience, facility owners expect a strong improvement in the happiness and satisfaction of the residents and their families.

Honors, Recognitions, and Distinctions – A Strong Tradition at Sharon Lane

Our attention to our core philosophies is evident in the retention rate of our employees and in the recognitions we receive at the local, state, and national levels.

Our Department Director's longevity is an average of six years. The overall licensed nurse turnover per year is 26% compared to the industry average of 47%.

Our nursing assistant turnover per year is 36% compared to the industry average of 86%.

Sharon Lane has been recognized as a 2010 recipient of the *Bronze – Commitment to Quality* National Quality Award presented by the American Health Care Association and National Center for Assisted Living (AHCA/NCAL), a trade organization with approximately 11,000 members nationwide. This year 701 nursing homes and assisted living communities from across the nation applied for the Bronze Quality Award, and Sharon Lane was one of 450 organizations to receive the award.

Implemented by AHCA/NCAL in 1996, the National Quality Award Program is based on the core values and criteria of the *Malcolm Baldrige National Quality Award Program. It* provides a pathway for providers of long term and post-acute care services to journey towards performance excellence. Facilities begin their quality journey where they are asked to develop an organizational profile, including vision and mission statements, an awareness of their environment and customers' expectations. Applicants are also asked to demonstrate their ability to improve the process of care giving. The applications are reviewed by Examiners who have received special training to qualify as judges for the award program.

"The commitment to quality designated by this award is a key step to developing systematic, sustainable, person-centered care and services," stated Bruce Yarwood, President and CEO of AHCA/NCAL. "We congratulate Sharon Lane on this achievement."

Sharon Lane is proud of its accomplishments, yet never loses its desire for continued improvement in the quality of life for its residents and their families. It is that attention to the greater good that allows Sharon Lane to be on the leading edge of national recognition standards:

Sharon Lane is a 4-star rated facility on a 5-star national rating scale.

Sharon Lane currently recognized no deficiency in the federal and state surveys. Sharon Lane is recognized as one of 13 of a combined 357 skilled nursing facilities in the State of Kansas in 2008 to obtain this designation.

Sharon Lane celebrates its Nursing Assistant of the year-Sharon Stauch, 2009, honored by the Kansas Health Care Association. Through her selfless efforts to provide the best care for our residents, Sharon gives testament to the unparalleled quality of service our nurses give to the residents and their families. Sharon sees her position as one of privilege, not of obligation, and that is the inherent difference in mindset.

Angela Moore, RN, BSN, LNHA, was honored with the Administrator of the Year designation from the Kansas Health Care Association. Recognized as a future leader in   long term care, Angela participated in the American Health Care Association/National Center for Assisted Living's "Future Leaders of Long Term Care in America" symposium held in Washington, DC, in 2009. Angela continues to demonstrate her leadership potential and aptitude for representing the interests of long term care providers at the state and national levels, with an emphasis on quality management, customer satisfaction, and leadership.

In October of 2008, Sharon Lane Health Services received the rare and honorable distinction from the State of Kansas as being a Deficiency-Free Facility, evidencing no deficiencies relative to patient care, quality of life, or patient safety. Sharon Lane Health Services was one of nine facilities out of 347 nursing homes in the state to receive this distinction.

With its fifty-plus years of service to the community, Sharon lane is a family-owned facility that specializes in providing intimate long-term care or short-term rehabilitative services for seniors.

History of Harry Baum

It has been an impressive and distinguished career for Dr. Harry Baum, and one that does not seem to be ending any time soon. With a Doctorate in Adult Education and Administration; a long-term care administrator's license in Kansas and in Missouri; and over three decades of experience in the long term care industry, Dr. Baum is a force with which to be reckoned as he continually gains new ground in the health care arena.

Because he has resided within the Kansas City area for most of his life, Dr. Baum is well-acquainted with the community. His extensive experience in health care began in St. Louis, Missouri in the Occupational Therapy Program through Washington University. While in that capacity, Dr. Baum wrote grants, co-taught classes in anatomy and physiology and worked with occupational therapy students in the area of rehabilitation. He continued in the health care and rehabilitation industry with the Saint Mary's hospital group, serving as the director of their educational programming for staff, residents, families, and the community in their rehabilitation hospital in St. Louis.

Building on his already solid career in health care, Dr. Baum then assumed the role of administrator in a 120 bed facility in the suburbs of St. Louis. While in this position, within 18 months, he increased the occupancy of the facility from 56 residents to 120 with a waiting list, all through dedicated marketing efforts and involvement within the community. Simultaneously, he brought the facility into compliance with all state regulations.

Because of his tireless efforts and dedication to the facility, the holding company was able to sell it at a 35% profit. Once the sale was completed, Dr. Baum maintained his association with the company through a variety of roles, including that of consultant administrator of a 220 bed facility in St. Louis. He also directed the establishment of four comprehensive outpatient rehabilitation facilities that provided physical therapy, occupational therapy, social service, and pastoral care for the nursing home residents.

Dr. Baum's next career step brought him back to the Kansas City area where he became the Administrator of a 240 bed facility at 120th and Wornall Road. While in this role, he increased the occupancy from 170 residents to 198 during the first year, and 228 residents during the next six months. In addition, he developed a 24 bed special care Alzheimer's unit.

This success was not to go unnoticed, and Dr. Baum was then recruited to the role of Executive Director at Cosada Delmar Retirement facility in North Kansas City, a 180 bed skilled nursing center. True to his track record, Dr. Baum took the occupancy from 135 residents to 176 in his first year and maintained those efforts for over four years.

When the company was sold in 1989, Dr. Baum spent the next ten years as a partner with one of the former owners of Cosada Delmar. He was responsible for the total operations of the partnership which began with a 25% ownership of a 180 bed skilled nursing facility. Over the next decade, Dr. Baum grew the company into three facilities consisting of 585 beds in Kansas, Missouri, and Arizona and simultaneously created his own consulting company. After selling his interest in the partnership in 2000, Dr. Baum and his family purchased Sharon Lane in 2001.

Dr. Baum's academic career consists of a B.S. in Education from the University of Kansas (1967); an M.S. in Administration and Supervision from the University of Kansas (1973); and a Doctorate in Education with an emphasis on Administration and Supervision from the University of Kansas (1980).

In addition to his vast experience within the health care industry, Dr. Baum also held positions in education as a teacher and in academic programs in various school districts within the metropolitan Kansas City area early on in his career. He and his wife, Connie, have four children and seven grandchildren.

Chapter One: Management Vs. Leadership

Are you a leader or a manager?

If you are a leader, are you also a manager? Leadership is one facet of management. A successful manager does possess the attributes of a strong leader. There is a marked difference, however, between a leader and a manager. The main goal of a manager is to make the most of the organization's output through attention to administrative details. In an effort to do this, a manager must be capable of organization, planning, staffing, directing, and controlling. Leadership is just one aspect of this modality.

Managers tend to think incrementally. Leaders think more radically – they see the big picture. Managers follow the rules of the book. Leaders are unafraid to color outside the context of those lines. Leaders rely more on intuition and tend to run on the fuel of emotion more than managers do. A true leader will stand out as being different. A true leader will question assumption and grow suspicious of tradition. Leaders make decisions based on truth and understanding as opposed to prejudice. They have a real desire for innovative thinking and implementation. Instead of trying to control others, leaders must make good use of their abilities to employ vision, implement strategy, and pursue goals.

When it comes to groups, the tendency is tosubscribe one's loyalty to the leader as opposed to the manager. This loyalty is generated by the leader taking responsibility by taking the blame when things go wrong; by celebrating group achievements, even the minor ones, and by giving credit where it is justly due. The leader will take the initiative to highlight the successes of a team by using charts, graphs, and entertaining presentations. It takes a true observer and sensitive individual to be a leader. A leader knows his team and will develop mutual confidence within that structure.

A leader is followed while a manager rules. People will naturally follow a leader by choice, whereas a manager must be obeyed. A manager may have been given his position essentially through years of hard work, dedication, and loyalty to his company, and not necessarily as a result of true leadership qualities. A leader may not have any organizational skills, but possesses a vision that genuinely unites those behind him.

Management is usually a structure of key players who are highly experienced within their given field. They are typically those individuals who have worked their way up through company ranks. A manager is familiar with each layer of the system and how those layers operate. A manager possesses solid technical knowledge.

A leader, however, can be a new arrival to the company. He is bold and determined, bearing fresh, new ideas and concepts, yet may be lacking in specific experience and wisdom.

In short, managing and leading are two different ways of organizing people. A manger will use a formal, more rational methodology, and a leader is guided by passion and emotion.

For those individuals working in the thick of it, an educated and experienced perspective comes through. For Connie Baum, Director of Nursing at Sharon Lane, there is a distinct difference between leaders and managers.

"Managers get paid to get things done," she noted. "And this is usually within a strict budget. Managers have to plan with more details. Leaders have followers and a vision of where the organization is headed."

This begs the question: Can a charge nurse be both a leader and a manager? If so, how?

What is apparently lacking in the nursing school curriculum is an emphasis on teaching leadership skills, problem solving skills, and decision-making skills. The inherent problem with nursing schools is that they truly do not emulate real life. The nursing school programs tend to focus on a task-oriented education, leaving holes and gaps in areas of real need.

When someone lacks the ability to lead, there are certain attributes missing.

Traits of an effective leader

How does one become the proverbial Pied Piper? The success of a leader is due largely in part to the willingness of the people to follow him or her without feeling as if they are over-managed or obligated to do so. Further, these followers, if you will, tend to have a greater degree of morale and claim more ownership in their jobs.

What are the defining attributes of an effective leader? For starters, a strong leader has solid overall character traits. They act with integrity at every turn, and when standing in the shadow of doubt, they always do the right thing. They are honest, truthful, and straightforward, never promising what they cannot deliver.

A strong leader has a solid work ethic. This does not necessarily mean he or she works 18 hour days. It speaks more to the efficiency by which he or she works during the hours of work. Of course, a strong leader is usually the first to arrive and the last to leave. It is easy for people to follow one who displays these attributes.

Leaders are passionate about what they do. They do not view their jobs as work at all. It is pleasurable for them. When they are faced with challenges, these are seen as opportunities. When stumbling blocks present themselves, a strong leader will simply turn those over into stepping stones to greater success. Leaders thrive on a consistent "whatever it takes" mentality. As such, they are operating on positive energy and enthusiasm that can be richly infectious to those around them. When a person is passionate about what he or she does, the results are usually nothing short of spectacular.

A sad fact of leadership at times is one's tendency to be reactive to situations instead of proactive. This can create more frustrations for team members and can stir up unnecessary negative energy throughout the team. It may also contribute to work activities that are of no-value and that might even generate additional costs.

An effective leader, then, is one who is proactive in situations. He or she anticipates a situation before it becomes an actual problem. This greatly reduces frustrations among the staff and is one sure-fire way to increase credibility as a leader.

Communication is an art not readily lost on a strong and effective leader. It is important to keep the team informed through frequent and accurate information. An effective leader understands that the staff greatly influences the efficiency of an organization as a whole. Therefore, it is imperative for a leader to share information as pertains to individual performance, expectations of the organization, and the overall state of the business.

(Source to credit: UMKC The Bloch School of Management)

Chapter Two: Medical Model Vs. Patient Model

There is a vast difference between the operations of hospitals and the operations of long term care facilities. As far as the nursing structure goes between these two types of facilities, the hospitals represent a very vertical type of organization, supported by a host of layers. Long term care facilities, on the other hand, represent a largely horizontal modality. As such, with a decreased amount of layers, fewer employees are engaging in more tasks.

Nursing schools do a remarkable job in teaching their students the task-oriented skills. The students are taught the basic methodologies of nursing. What is lacking in the overall curriculum, in my mind, is a clear focus on the big picture. There needs to be an emphasis on management skills as a functioning modality of nursing. Students graduate from nursing school with a solid set of practical nursing skills, which is great, but what about management skills? These are an integral part of the job and something that needs to be explored on the academic level. A need for management skills within the field of nursing exists in both the management of time and in the management of people.

With typical management styles, there is the trend to focus on the negative, to hone in on the problems as opposed to working on the possible solutions. There needs to be a balance to that equation by incorporating the positive with education in order to make the unit run more efficiently and smoothly.

At Sharon Lane, we have three units and three shifts throughout a 24-hour period. Each unit has a charge nurse assigned to it.

When the nurses at Sharon Lane were asked what the five most critical factors are in managing a unit, their responses were unanimous:

1.) A charge nurse must set an example through a solid work ethic.
2.) A charge nurse must be involved with the staff.
3.) A charge nurse must set and maintain standards and not let the standards of care diminish. He or she must stay involved and not allow things to get sloppy.
4.) A charge nurse must effectively communicate with the staff and allow for a free-flow of communication. The staff needs to feel comfortable in bringing questions and problems to the charge nurse. There has to be an environment of give and take.

It is important to manage the staff by allowing them to make decisions on their own. As a manager, you cannot dictate everything to the staff. You have to learn to trust them. It is imperative that you communicate goals to the unit and that these goals require one to be self-reliant and that they also provide for cooperative management.

The nurses at Sharon Lane like to start each shift with a five minute stand-up meeting or go out and walk with each staff member individually.

The night shift is the most important shift in the rotation. It dictates the flow of the next day. If everything goes smoothly from the night shift into the day shift, the day shift enjoys a productive shift. On the contrary, if the night shift has been sloppy or unproductive in the use of its time, the day shift must take up the slack, therefore losing necessary focus and key productivity time.

The nurse manager must create a list for what needs to be done, but there has to exist a certain sort of flexibility within those lists. Good management skills are the same as family management skills. You must be consistent. You must set goals and standards, and the boundaries must by clearly known and understood.

The Baby Boomers are facilitating the shift from the medical model to the patient model. As they enter the nursing home facilities, they have a desire to be in charge of their own decisions. They are unaccustomed to being told what to do and when to do it. Their independent attitudes are creating a need to move from the medical model to the social model. As such, those of us in the long term care industry have to be aware of people and their preferences. Patients tend to be more agreeable when they feel as if they have choices to make in matters of their personal care. The philosophy is simple: Just be nice to people. Have awareness. As a nurse, you still have to get your work accomplished, but you have to maintain that overall focus on the patient. However, as patients enter a nursing home facility, they have to be aware that it is not a place wherein they will receive continual one-on-

one time with a nurse. If someone is expecting that one-on-one care or round-the-clock supervision, then they are better off hiring an in-home care provider. Bear in mind, however, that can be expensive and challenging!

Chapter Three: Inspire To Motivate

How to get your team to take more ownership!

Sometimes all it takes is a bit of healthy change within an organization to heighten motivation, inspire a stronger work ethic, and make efficient use of one's time.

In order to implement changes, it has to be evident that everyone benefits. If employees see no benefits in the changes for them, they most likely won't jump on board. They need to know that in giving their greatest efforts to the change, that the benefits will be mutual. They will recognize if they are being exploited for their ideas. Everyone from the cleaning crews to the company's CEO needs to be mutually supportive. Even the greatest pep talks in the world will fail if the employees do not feel appreciated.

Be sure to publicly acknowledge and recognize any fresh, new ideas and achievements. This builds morale and promotes healthy change. When it comes to praise, formality does not have to be the mode of the day. If made a part of your daily communication, verbal compliments are far more effective. If you want to celebrate an employee's success, send out an e-mail to the entire department. Better yet, buy that individual lunch if he or she comes up with a truly inspired idea. Even small rewards make big impressions. When you show that you truly appreciate an employee's contribution, the motivation you receive from that person in return is unparalleled.

As a manager, you cannot be all talk and no action. You are the number one role model for every employee whom you supervise, and this needs to be evident in your actions. Come up with some of your own ideas, no matter how off-the-wall they might seem, if only to show that no idea is a bad one.

Leave an open door for feedback. Great ideas don't necessarily stem from isolation. They come from a supportive environment. Encourage your staff to communicate with you if they are getting the support they need to do their jobs effectively. Make yourself available to listen and give guidance. Practice the art of communication by actually listening to what your staff is saying, and, in some cases, repeat it back to them so they know you are truly hearing what they have to say.

Everyone wants to know that what they do matters. Explain to each staff member exactly how his or her role and individual performance fits into and affects the company's overall goals. This will allow them to understand how new ideas can have a lasting and positive impact on the success of the company.

As a manager, you need to show enthusiasm for your job. You have a choice to either make your shift feel like endless hours of drudgery, or you can make it feel like just a few quick hours of pleasure. You make the call. When your employees see your enthusiasm, it quickly becomes contagious.

Show your staff that you trust them and their abilities. Ask for their ideas. This boosts morale exponentially. Bear in mind, however, that if you stifle their enthusiasm and ignore their ideas, morale will plummet. Be open and honest, as well. If you truly believe that a suggested idea will not work, tell that person, but beware of destroying their self-confidence and self-esteem in the process. You will gain respect from that individual, as it will be evident that you are willing to speak the truth.

What is accepted as office behavior is learned by watching the boss. It is up to you to maintain a positive and upbeat persona. Exude enthusiastic energy. Teach your employees to stay productive, supporting each other, and this will allow for a continual flow of healthy change and inspired ideas.

(Source: http://www.allbusiness.com/human-resources/employee-development/2975055-1.html)

Chapter Four: Lead By Design

In evaluating management and leadership roles, is there really a difference? While the two do go hand-in-hand, they are quite different.

According to Bethany Spilde, a social media strategist, trainer, and leadership expert in Kansas City, management is an organizational function that focuses on getting things done through the management of subordinates (employees), time, and resources. Leadership, on the other hand, is a very important quality/asset that focuses on uniting and inspiring people towards visions of the future.

Leaders are typically focused on the future/vision/change. They act in a capacity to lead people, have followers through displayed charisma and passion. Leaders are achievers and risk-takers. They create and set the direction, often taking the road less traveled. They command loyalty, are courageous, have earned the trust of their followers, and are guided by intuition.

Managers are more focused on organizing, planning (details), managing work, incorporating stability, having authority (formal), dealing with subordinates (employees), are focused on results (getting things done), work to eliminate risk, and usually have experience (earned position in the company). Their goals are more short-term in nature, using efficient processes and existing paths to get the desired results.

This begs the question: Can a person be both a leader and a manager? Absolutely, notes Bethany.

"A manager who is also a leader is the one who is most effective at the job and in dealing with people. Managing "encouraged" people who are willing to follow that person towards a vision, with a specific plan in place. That is what leads to successful business. In other words, you obtain the best of both worlds."

Bethany would even argue that a company could have management without leadership, but it would not be as passionate and rewarding. It would simply be just work. It is hard to have leadership without having management, however.

Inspiring, motivating, and encouraging employees are critical tasks for a leader, but how is that done effectively? While it certainly depends on the type of leader or manager and the culture of the company and its employees, there are a variety of ways to do this. The bottom line is to show the employees (followers) that you care about them. Encourage them to excel and use their natural strengths and interest to achieve that bigger goal and vision. By creating a positive work environment where the employees are valued and can be heard, people will feel a sense of motivation and will most likely produce their best work. It is up to the leader to find ways to promote healthy minds, bodies, and spirits.

In short, a leader is followed. A manager "rules."

Chapter Five: Manage Your Time

Formerly a CNA prior to working at Sharon Lane, Stephanie Sweeten, RN, worked in a nursing home as well as in acute care through her employment with a nursing agency. She has been employed at Sharon Lane for three years and is now their Assistant Director of Nursing.

In her new role, Stephanie has quickly learned the qualities an exceptional nursing manager needs.

"First of all," she explained, "a nursing manager needs to be well-organized and highly confident in decision-making skills. When crises arise, it is crucial to maintain a sense of calm. If you are calm, then your patients and staff will be calm. Be aware of everything. Don't just focus on the small details."

Stephanie supervises about 50 people, although not all at one time. Her main focus is continually on what is best for the residents/patients at Sharon Lane. She also stressed that it is important to be aware of the patient's family members, too.

Time management plays a huge role in the job of a nurse manager, and Stephanie has taken copious mental notes on this issue.

"Always come to work prepared," she said. "If you have to, arrive early. Start your day with the most critical work first and then prioritize from there. Learn to delegate any tasks that you can and be sure to follow-up on those later on to make sure they have been done."

It also goes without saying that you need to work hard during your shift. Stay focused. Get the work done.

Stephanie understands that balancing time and tasks means being persuasive in your approach with the patients. She emphasizes to try what works best for them and then remain flexible. Flexibility will be your friend. Nothing is exact. Be sure to delegate matters to the CNAs and to the on-coming shift.

"Delegating work to the on-coming shift should not represent a problem unless you are in the habit of continually passing something on to them and have set a pattern for this behavior. The delegating of which I am speaking is in reference to non-critical orders. Not something you should have done in the first place."

Now with quality experience behind her in the nursing field, Stephanie does agree that the academic experience for nurses stresses a vast amount of technical things, losing sight of the leadership and management elements that are just as important for the nurse. She believes that nursing schools should make a management experience for the students towards the end of their schooling wherein they have an opportunity to manage their peers. Through that experience, they can find their weaknesses and strengths. They can take turns managing each other before they are thrown out onto the floor in a real life nursing situation. Through this simulated practice, they can assess what they need to work on and find room to grow. Stephanie truly believes this is the management component that should be incorporated into the curriculum at every nursing school. This could also be incorporated at the job site with the cooperation of other charge nurses and nursing management. Simulated role playing and counseling by experienced nurses could be of great value.

Chapter Six: Lend An Ear; Recognize A Voice

Conflict Management

Does anyone truly enjoy conflict, personally or professionally? Not really, but it is a common side effect when it comes to managing people. While some simply choose to avoid conflict, the emphasis should remain on resolving it. Rare is the work place where conflict is not common.

There was once an ancient philosopher who pontificated, "Everyone should be quick to listen, slow to speak, and slow to become angry." Despite the fact that we all have two ears, research has shown that we only operate at about 25% efficiency when using them.

A common cause of conflict stems from the fact that we do not listen well, or carefully enough, either to the content or to the emotions associated with that content. In short there are three hurdles that prevent us from fully engaging our listening skills: presumption, impatience, and pride.

When we do not effectively listen while on the job, the results can be in the form of miscommunication, errors, decreased productivity and morale, increased turnover, and the loss of customers.

When you are listening to someone, you have to know and understand why you are listening. You should also clue yourself into to the non-verbal elements of communication. Focus on gestures and body language. When you are listening, organize what you are hearing through observation, note-taking, and reflective listening. A good skill to employ is to repeat back what you heard to the person expressing it. This will (1) let that person know you truly are listening and (2) clear up any miscommunication if the message is not fully understood.

Give your complete attention to the individual speaking to you. If you cannot do so, please advise them and make time for when you can genuinely listen to his or her concerns. Keep distractions at bay, and remember that the best tools to use when listening really are your ears. Resist the temptation to render advice, make predictions, or ask questions, and above all, do not interrupt. Nothing disrupts the flow of clear and concise communication like interruptions do. And, as poetic as it might sound, listen with your mind as well as with your heart.

Chapter Seven: So You're A Supervisor... Now What?

Connie Baum heralds the position of Director of Nursing at Sharon Lane. When it comes to the education of nurses, what she deems as lacking in the academic arena is a focus on leadership skills, problem solving skills, and decision making skills. There is no emphasis on future thinking and thought processes in that regard. An individual graduates from nursing school and is now technically a nurse, but what exactly does that mean? What does it entail?

Connie indicated that within the four-year curriculum to earn an RN degree, there is some instruction on leadership, but it is minimal, at best. She stresses that those who do grasp it tend to come by it naturally. Others may think, however, that in order to be a good leader, you have to be loud. That is a big misconception. One course on leadership skills in school is simply not enough.

While certain personalities are distinct in the nursing field, most people generally think of nurses as caring. Connie stresses that some nurses are quiet, some may be loud, and some just do not have solid leadership skills. They cannot get people to follow them. They do not understand how to effectively listen, nor do they take the time to build relationships and a solid foundation of trust between them and their staff. Charge nurses and supervisors must learn to openly communicate with their unit and get constant feedback.

So, what is lacking most of the time in a charge nurse's or supervisor's ability to lead people? According to Angela Moore, Administrator at Sharon Lane, the motivation is just not there. The individual is unable to see a vision of what they need to do, of the ability they do have, and where they want the unit to go. There is a lack of building team work skills. At Sharon Lane, Angela emphasizes that the basics are continually taught to new hires. The supervisors must let their employees know the expectations for each shift. At the beginning of each shift, they need to sit down with the staff and indicate what is going on, what needs to be done, and then they have to follow-up with that communication by checking in consistently throughout the shift, making sure to thank the staff for all of their hard work along the way.

In most nursing school curriculums, organizational skills, time management skills, and even the simple elements of preparing daily "to do" lists are not taught. While the seasoned nurses may do this, those who come right out of school typically do not. They may have one to two patients in a hospital setting and then suddenly they are faced with five, 10, or even 30 patients and five to six staff members directly underneath them. Then what?

Under these types of conditions, most supervisors will tend to shut down and focus in on the tasks instead. The presumption is, if they are not getting the task done, they are not doing their job. What they are failing to recognize is their real responsibility rests in those 30 patients on their floor. They are responsible for 30 lives...not just tasks! School is one arena, but in the real world, it is a completely different ball game.

In fact, in about 50% of cases or more, a nurse will not grasp the full effect of this until he or she is on the second, and quite possibly the third, job. Unless they are quick learners, it usually takes two to three jobs to get better and to fully understand the need for leadership skills, communication skills, organizational skills, and time management skills. In short, it is a two-three year "training period" outside of school. Why not teach this in school to reduce that gap?

In a hospital environment, a nurse supervisor deals with fewer patients than in a long term care facility. In a hospital, one is dealing with an illness and may just be assigned to a total of five patients. They may have to supervise just one aide. The nursing environment in a hospital is somewhat less stressful and considerably different than in a long-term care facility. If one truly wants to understand what nursing is all about, then working in a long term care facility can provide that understanding, and then some.

In a long term care environment, a nurse has more responsibility. Sure, there is still technical knowledge involved, but at this level, the issues are more complex, and there are more patients/families and more duties to manage. The nurses in a long term care facility are the extended arm of the physician, who is usually not on the premises. In a hospital, a nurse can generally converse with the doctor if there is a problem. That is not the situation in nursing homes.

In a hospital setting, the nurse has more access to the physicians, and it is the physicians who make most of the decisions. In long term care situations, the nurses must make most of the decisions and pair those decisions with good management skills and organizational skills. It is an all-encompassing process.

For those charge nurses and supervisors working in long term care, it is imperative that they communicate not only to their own team, but to the oncoming shift as well. Good communication skills are essential to the survival of the unit as a whole.

At Sharon Lane, we provide a significant amount of education for our nurses. We teach them how to gain the necessary skills from the start to become better leaders. We stress the importance of this. According to Connie, the Director of Nursing at Sharon Lane, if a nurse wants to learn these skills, it is important that he or she works for an employer who recognizes the need for them. The nurses must admit to themselves that they do not know this and then understand it is okay to ask. In fact, it is encouraged. There is no shame in asking, "I'm not sure how to do this, so can you help me?" when inquiring of a supervisor. It is the responsibility of the supervisor to provide the answers and assistance. If not the supervisor, then find the answer from the Director of Nursing or the Assistant Director of Nursing. There are not a lot of layers within a long term care environment, so it is important to know of whom you should ask these questions. As an employer, it is our responsibility to provide the answers and resources. We have a 50% commitment to that end, and the employee has a 50% commitment to ask and to learn. If the Director of Nursing or the Administrator of Nursing is not available, inquire of someone who has been around and seems successful within the organization. A new nurse needs to be proactive in resolving what he or she does not know.

The problem is that most nurses are afraid to ask, for fear it will get them into trouble or make them look foolish. If you have a question and the person to provide the answer is not available, contact that person and make an appointment to speak with him or her. Find a way to get hold of someone who can help. It's that easy. Don't let fear or embarrassment become obstacles to your success as a nurse.

It is true that administrators and supervisors get busy, and because of that, they may fail to ask if the new nurses need help and may fail to follow-up. Supervisors must not allow this to happen!

In a sense, being a supervisor is akin to being a coach, and your coaching sessions with your employees can be spontaneous in nature or take the form of a   planned meeting. This is a challenging skill for many supervisors. Coaching allows you to create a platform wherein the employee creates a solution to a problem or situation. It alleviates the need for you, as the supervisor, to provide advice or tender a solution for the employee. It gives the employee both ownership and accountability. Through effective questioning, you can empower your employees to proactively manage their individual performances.

As a supervisor/coach, you can work with each employee to identify any obstacles that can impede an employee's ability to fulfill certain goals. These could include external obstacles, such as a busy schedule, limited resources, ambiguous or incomplete information, and interactions with others. It can include the internal obstacles, such as fear of failure, lack of confidence, lingering self-doubt, an unwillingness to change, an inability to make decisions, or a misunderstanding of expectations.

As a coach, you begin to foster an employee's awareness and understanding of his or her role and responsibility, allowing that employee to take ownership of ideas, actions, and goals, all of which are crucial to good performance.

It takes patience and effort to conduct these "coaching sessions," as well as some practice, but it is worth the endeavor. Your employees will respond favorably and positively to your commitment to their success. Giving continuous feedback shows that you are dedicated to building a positive and trusting relationship with your employees and shows you are willing to assist them in improving their overall performance. In addition, it allows you to improve your performance as a supervisor! This creates a win-win situation for all!

As a supervisor, you must engage in the orientation period for each new hire. This orientation period, however, is not a one-day affair. It can be several days, several weeks, or even months. It all depends on the employee and his or her comfort level with the position. Each new employee must be confident and feel capable of engaging in all of the responsibilities of the job. This includes knowing when to take breaks, where to get a drink of water, and even where to put a coffee cup. They must feel confident in all aspects of the job, no matter how small.

A charge nurse's responsibility is to monitor the orientation period and help make the employee feel comfortable and give them the opportunity to ask questions if they do not understand or know something. They should feel comfortable in being able to approach the supervisor if they are uncertain or if something is wrong. LISTENING is a vital aspect of the charge nurse's role. The charge nurse must watch what is happening out on the floor and recognize all clues, both verbal and non-verbal, that are coming from the staff. Does someone have a scowl on her face? Is someone not particularly friendly or not laughing and engaging with others? If something appears to be wrong, then find out what it is and solve the problem. If you are task-oriented with your head down at your desk and tending to all of the detailed tasks at hand, you will miss out on what is going on. You cannot see the big picture from a microscopic level. This is true not only during the orientation process, but in the day-to-day operations as well.

When you are so task-oriented, you tend to ignore the emotional aspect of situations. This is a big hurdle to overcome with nurses in general. You have to learn to back off of the tasks at times and see the big picture. Ask yourself: How is the unit working? How is the unit being managed? Are all systems and processes efficient? Are staff members helping each other? Are they verbally communicating with each other?

This is one of the biggest areas of concern with charge nurses. Their main focus tends to be on the documentation, the medications, and the charts, calling the doctors, and dealing with the paperwork. Sure, those are elements of the job, but if you are not getting out on the floor and observing and interacting, then you are ignoring the big picture and, quite frankly, the attention to true patient care.

When you, as the charge nurse, get out on the floor, do you walk with your head down and blinders on, focused on all the minute technical details of your job, or are you walking with your head up, your eyes wide open, and engaging with those in the hall? Are you seeing everything and observing what needs to be handled immediately? Are you assessing potential problems? Are you observing if the unit is nice and comfortable and that all of the residents are getting their needs met?

Another issue of concern is the call light. Too many times, with task-oriented mentality, nurses get bogged down in their paperwork, and they literally ignore that call light. They remain completely unaware that there is a problem outside of their little area because they are too busy taking notes, writing, and documenting. This is where you need to learn to sit back, be aware, and really observe what is going on so that you can solve the bigger problems that will utilize your other skills. If you see that a problem exists, you can get up and take care of it. By solving the bigger problems at hand, this can greatly reduce the overall stress of managing the unit.

Sometimes it just takes small steps to produce big impacts. Take the time to go visit a patient. Talk to them. Ask them how they are doing. Tell them that you were thinking about them and wanted to see if there was anything they needed. On the way down the hall to visit that patient, look around. See if anyone needs anything. Are your aides happy? Ask how they are doing. Compliment them. Find something they are doing well and tell them they are doing a good job. Show that you truly care. The return on that investment of your time will reap exponential gains.

Closing Comments

Are you following the leader or leading the followers?

As a true leader, you must be honest, respectful, and knowledgeable in your role, and you must possess the confidence in your ability to fulfill your role, effectively communicate with your staff, and openly ask for their opinions. Always remember it is the people you are supervising or your followers who determine if you are a good leader or not. Their vision of you as good or ineffective will determine if they follow you or not. If they are going to follow someone, then that someone must earn their respect and trust.

Remember that different employees require different models of leadership. A new employee, for example, may need a bit more supervision than a seasoned employee. If you have an employee with little motivation, then that particular individual may require a different approach than the employee that is driven and motivated. You have to understand your employees to determine your most effective leadership style.

(Commentary from Connie Baum, RN, MSN, Director of Nursing at Sharon Lane Health Services)

"Don't Tell ME What to Do!"

That sentiment tends to reflect the attitudes and opinions of many employees today. They often want to be part of something bigger than the menial day-to-day tasks and chores. They want to be involved in solving the problems, not just being told what to do to correct those problems.

To successfully motivate employees, you have to involve them and make them feel as if they are truly a part of the problem-solving, solution-oriented process. Your employees must believe in you in order for this to effectively work. Sincerity and authenticity must be readily transparent in your actions and in your defined goals, paired with consistency in your decision-making process. Keep in mind that your staff will always be a part of everything you do and that you need them to maintain complete faith and trust in you. If they do not, then they will not completely buy into the goals, and thus fall short of reaching them.

Employees need to know that you really do care about them, their goals, and their situations. Don't just give them lip service. For example, if an employee who is reliable and sincerely cares about the health and well-being of the patients and is a quality employee, confides in me that his car broke down and he does not have the funds at the moment to fix it, I will try to help him solve the problem by communicating to administration his situation for the possibility of an advance in wages worked.

If another employee shares a personal struggle and asks for help, I will listen to her and offer my help in any way I can. This sends the message that I truly do care and that I am investing my time and energy into her. This establishes that bond of trust and respect and shows that I do care about her. In turn, she begins to sense that she can count on me to listen and help her when I can. This is true for all of your employees.

Sadly, many of the employees with whom we work in long-term care have had past experiences with those in their lives who have let them down in some capacity or another. They feel betrayed and sense that there is no one in whom they can trust and confide. It takes time to build their loyalty and trust, but when you do, the avenues for motivation and inspiration are wide open. Goals are more readily met. The employees are happier and genuinely want to do a good job. They become excited about being more involved in their jobs and in the team environment, giving their input and seeing some of their ideas lead to positive action, change, and results.

(Contributed by Angela Moore, Administrator, Sharon Lane Health Services)

NOTES:

NOW WHAT? PUTTING THEORY INTO PRACTICE

So, you have come this far! What's next? How do you put what you have learned into practice? The team of experts at Sharon Lane Health Services has provided you solid ideas and practical applications to everyday work place problems and situations. These next several pages will direct you as to how to put what you have learned into practice.

Making a Decision

So...what can you do when you have a decision to make? Do you flip a coin? Do you consult a psychic? I doubt either of those methods will render useful results. However, here is a series of defining steps that can make the road to a decision a smoothly-paved one:

1.) You have to define the problem first.
2.) Then you must identify the limiting factors.
3.) Be prepared to develop potential alternatives.
4.) Analyze those alternatives.
5.) From those alternatives, select the best one.
6.) Confidently implement your decision.
7.) Follow-up on that decision by establishing an evaluation system.

No matter the depth and width of the decision to be made, this process must take place in order for good decisions to be made and executed.

Dealing with Conflicting Demands without Going Crazy

There will be those days when you are faced with the seemingly daunting challenge of wrestling with two conflicting demands. In order to effectively deal with those demands, you have to understand the following priorities in order to establish which concern takes precedence:

1.) Safety
2.) Courtesy
3.) Show
4.) Efficiency

Items one and four are clear-cut. Show and courtesy are somewhat vague. Show is what relates to everything that makes a sensory impression. It is a matter of presentation, or how well an area "shows" to a patient. Courtesy is how well they are treated with attention, respect, and a caring attitude. How much you allow their opinion to be heard concerning their care, wants, and needs. For those Baby Boomers that will soon segue into long-term care facilities and rehabilitation centers in the coming decades, this list of priorities will conform to their expectations and demands.

The main criteria for determining admission or discharge to and from a facility focus on the safety of the patient. If the patient cannot be safe in any other environment, then they will be admitted to the facility. If, on the other hand, they can be safe either at home or in a lesser level of care, then they can be confidently discharged.

While it can be a challenge to effectively prioritize the priorities listed above, perhaps it is best to recognize them as almost equal priorities, not on a ladder, but more on a slightly inclined stair step. In other words, if patient satisfaction is your primary objective, then all of those priorities listed above must be followed and in the order given. Traditionally in the medical model in post-acute settings, efficiency is at the top of the list of priorities. The staff must get all tasks accomplished efficiently at the staff's convenience.

Not commonly seen in post-acute settings is putting courtesy second only to safety. Everything is given equal lip service, except efficiency is at the top. Nothing else is given priority over the other. This creates confusion and a significant variation in courtesy. **Thus, if patient satisfaction is to be a key for you, then the above priorities: safety, courtesy, show, and efficiency must be followed in your work with equal attention to each!**

Also: Be sure to investigate, identify, and tend to the true needs of each unique, specific patient. Be creative. Color outside of the lines and think outside of the box.

Be sure to investigate, identify, and tend to the true needs of each unique, specific employee in your charge. Be creative. Color outside of the lines and think outside of the box.

(The referenced ideas were from "If Disney Ran Your Hospital," by Fred Lee, Copyright 2004.)

**Speak your mind and enjoy the results!
Communication is key!**

When dealing with staff members, if you don't verbally express to them what your expectations of them are, then they will be left in the dark. Be precise and concise in what it is you expect them to do during their shift. Be sure to provide this clear communication at the beginning of each shift. Be sure to engage in follow-up communications with your staff by arranging specific times for them to check in with you during the day, such as two hours into the shift, before going on any breaks, and before leaving for the day.

Set clear time frames for when you expect certain tasks to be performed, such as the taking of vital signs, bathing, toileting, etc. Make sure each staff member informs you of when these specific tasks have been completed.

Don't spend your time hovered over your desk during the entire shift. Go on rounds. Your staff must know and anticipate that you are following up on what you requested them to do.

The most important element of communication is to thank each staff member and sincerely express your gratitude for what they have accomplished at the end of their shift.

(Commentary from Connie Baum, RN, MSN, Director of Nursing at Sharon Lane Health Services)

How to handle a not-so-cooperative employee:

If it is professional behavior and attitudes you desire of your employees, you must first embrace that quality yourself. You are the role model for them. How can you expect something from them if you don't exhibit the same behavior?

When dealing with an insubordinate employee, never do so in front of others. There are those select few who crave an audience so that the other employees can perhaps view them as tough and incapable of being told what to do by a superior.

Example scenario:

A CNA arrives for her scheduled shift 25 minutes late. As her supervisor, you approach the CNA and indicate, "I see that you are 25 minutes late today. Is there something that caused you to be late?" The CNA casually responds that she just overslept, and you respond to this excuse by noting that you and her fellow staff members expect her to be on time, as it is one of the key responsibilities of her role. The CNA then turns to an attitude of defensiveness, bursting out, "Can I help it if my alarm clock didn't go off? What do you expect me to do? Why are you on my case? I don't have to put up with this. I don't have to put up with this garbage. In fact, I am going to report you, as you have no right to speak to me in that manner, and you never say anything to anyone else who shows up late!"

An appropriate response from you to this tirade should resemble this:

"I need you to come into the office so we can talk." You should never address the employee in front of others and never counsel them without a witness. Once you are in a private setting, you must take control of the situation. You must inform the employee that she is being insubordinate and that this is unacceptable behavior and will not, under any circumstances, be tolerated.

If she responds genuinely apologetic and realizes she was wrong and promises not to exhibit such unprofessional behavior again, then provide her with a written warning following your facility policy if the behavior should occur again.

However, if the response from the insubordinate employee is negative, then you must ask her to clock out and go home and that she cannot return until approval from her supervisor. If she refuses to follow your directions and continues to be loud and disruptive, call the police and have her promptly escorted from the premises.

NEVER, EVER...under any circumstances.....lay your hands on the employee for any reason.

(Commentary from Connie Baum, RN, MSN, Director of Nursing at Sharon Lane Health Services)

Practical Examples of Leadership and Management

The following represent two scenarios that provide insightful examples of common situations within the field of long-term care nursing:

1.) Mrs. Smith's daughter, Jane, who is also her DPOA (durable power of attorney), is visiting today, and you are caught off-guard when she approaches you and begins to vocalize her frustrations with how you are supposedly not doing a good job in taking care of her mother. She wants to know why her mom is so lethargic, seems more confused than ever, and even mentioned something about having to take a new medication this morning. As the charge nurse, how will you effectively respond to this?

First of all, it is important to remain calm. If you become tense and agitated, bordering on defensive posture, then you will have an exceedingly more challenging time in resolving the conflict at hand. When you are approached by an upset family member or patient, always ensure you give them adequate time to express their concerns fully, without interrupting them. Genuinely listen to what they have to say. Body language is important here, as well. Do not stand with your arms crossed over your chest. Instead, relax your arms at your side, hands open, and palms slightly up. Give yourself an opportunity to evaluate the situation at hand and then validate how they feel by repeating back to them, as sincerely as possible, what they just explained to you.

Explain that Mrs. Smith has recently developed a urinary tract infection and began to take an antibiotic for it this morning. Unfortunately, since you have been off of this unit for the past week, you realize this information was not communicated to Mrs. Smith's daughter in a timely manner. Do not make excuses or place blame on your fellow team members. Instead, politely apologize for the lack of communication and begin to educate the family member on the changes that have taken place with the patient. You cannot change what has already occurred, but you can make a positive impact towards the remainder of their stay. Following the education given, offer the family member an opportunity to ask any questions or to clarify any further concerns. Then, make sure that Mrs. Smith's daughter is fully aware she can call or approach you in the future should she have any additional questions or concerns regarding her mother's plan of care. Hopefully, by the end of this interaction, you will have observed a change in her demeanor and will have cultivated a good rapport with her. In turn, she will most likely respect you and the manner in which you conducted yourself, leaving the avenue of communication open, positive, and easily accessible the next time.

2.) At the change of a shift, you notice that several nurse assistants at the nurse's station are bickering over the assignments for that day. As you approach them, you overhear one announce, "I am not working that hall again. You know Mrs. Jones will be on the light the entire night!" Then another one chimes in: "Well, I've never even worked that section before; I can't work with these people." As the charge nurse, how can you effectively handle the situation? Do you just ignore the comments?

Negativity in the work place is a vicious virus. It can spread like wild fire if not handled effectively. It only takes one individual to begin complaining, and, before you realize it, the entire team has become disgruntled about one thing or another. As a charge nurse, it is highly essential that you maintain a positive, team-centered approach. Ignoring the negative chatter of the employees you are managing will not resolve anything, but will only encourage a larger problem to develop.

It is important to direct and encourage the aides to support each other and to work together so that everyone can successfully care for the residents and get the assigned tasks completed by the end of the shift.

In regards to the CNA who does not want to work with certain residents because they are needy, direct that person to approach that particular resident at the beginning of the shift to let the patient know the CNA will be caring for her that evening and ask if there is anything the CNA can do for her while things are quiet. By addressing that patient first thing, the CNA can begin to meet the needs of that resident before the resident has to push her call light numerous times to get what she needs.

Further, encourage the other CNAs to jump in and take turns answering Mrs. Jones' call light, should she continue to have numerous needs that night, so that the aide can assist all of the residents to which she is assigned.

Have an experienced aide work closely with the aide using a buddy system, handling both aides' assignments. The experienced aide offers a review of each resident's needs, preferences, and care until the aide becomes familiar with all the residents. This way, all residents receive the correct care necessary and the new or less experienced CNA receives the education needed.

(Commentary from Stephanie Sweeten, RN, Assistant Director of Nursing at Sharon Lane Health Services)

How to Educate Your Staff on a Daily Basis

In a long-term care setting, time is a precious commodity. As such, you have to learn to make the most out of every single moment available to you. On most days, a charge nurse might not be able to find structured time to educate all of his or her CNAs in one lengthy setting, as they are all too busy caring for the residents. Thus, it is important that you learn to make the most of each moment and situation by bringing the teaching alongside each work experience. This is a kind of "educate-as-you-go-along" approach.

Instead of answering questions with a quick "yes" or "no," the charge nurse must take the opportunity at hand to educate his or her team members. That way, he or she is better prepared the next time around when they encounter that exact same situation. This makes the team member aware of the rationale behind the task in which he or she is involved.

(Commentary from Stephanie Sweeten, RN, Assistant Director of Nursing at Sharon Lane Health Services)

How You Can Effectively Increase Communication with Your Staff Daily

1.) Create and maintain a routine. Set expectations so your staff is fully aware of what is expected of them, not only for that day, but in the coming days, weeks, and months.
2.) Begin each day with a brief meeting to review and assign tasks.
3.) Ensure that you report any changes with residents and additional needs they might have outside of their normal routines.
4.) Make yourself fully available to your staff. If you are not available, approachable, or worse, if your staff cannot even find you, then they will begin to think that their input is not of value to you. As such, you have just cut yourself off from a wealth of information, as well as diminished your chances of growing a functional team.

Set specific time frames for tasks to be completed and then follow through on your end to make sure those tasks were done. If, for example, you indicate that a specific task is to be completed by 10 a.m., then you must follow-through and verify that it was, in fact, done....and done to your standards. If the members of your staff do not feel you really care about when things get accomplished or even how they get accomplished, then most likely they will not care, either. Additionally, should you find the completion of or the quality given to the task was not to your satisfaction, then address the staff member so that she can recognize that both elements are important to you. Without this in place, your direction and authority is compromised and is more or less a waste of time.

(Commentary from Stephanie Sweeten, RN, Assistant Director of Nursing at Sharon Lane Health Services)

Three Things a Charge Nurse Can Do Right Now to Motivate People

1.) Reward your staff with praise whenever possible. When people feel appreciated and recognized for what they do, especially from their superiors, they take the extra time to pay attention to the details and to return the favor in kind by recognizing someone else's extra efforts.
2.) Offer incentives to your staff whenever possible. Even small gestures can go a long way. For example, offer a candy bar to the aide who can successfully complete her monthly vital signs in the timeliest fashion.
3.) Keep the work environment as positive as possible. Employees do not function well, nor are they productive, in a negative environment. When surrounded with positive people and ideas, employees are more likely to enjoy their work, feel good about what they are doing, and make a bigger impact.

(Commentary from Stephanie Sweeten, RN, Assistant Director of Nursing at Sharon Lane Health Services)

Praising and Motivating Your Staff

What is praise, and why are so many people reluctant to praise someone, and likewise, why are so many people embarrassed to be on the receiving end of praise and compliments?

Let's face it. We live in a society with a scarcity of praise. You might be embarrassed to praise a staff member, and, more than likely, if you do praise a staff member, she might cower in embarrassment rather than soak in the compliments.

In an effort to consciously and sincerely praise my staff members, I have developed a simple tool for making sure that I praise people on a regular basis. All you need to do this is a positive attitude and a pocket of paper clips….or any collection of small items that won't take up too much space in your pockets, such as small coins, rubber bands, or buttons.

At the beginning of each day, I put several paper clips in my left pocket. Throughout the course of the day, I intentionally seek out staff members who are worthy of praise or who are doing something right, and then I compliment them on what they are doing. After I do that, I move one paper clip from the left pocket and place it into my right pocket. By the end of the day when all of my paper clips have been moved from my left pocket to my right pocket, I have assured myself that I have effectively, sincerely, and genuinely paid attention to my staff that day.

Notice my attention to the words "genuine" and "sincere." This tool for complimenting others is only effective when done from the heart. If your compliments sound empty and meaningless, perhaps even rehearsed or forced, then they will backfire on you. Don't do it just for the sake of doing it. Be authentic. If someone believes you mean what you say, they will fully appreciate it.

You can start this simple exercise by using just three paper clips and work up from there. This is a training exercise for yourself.

(Commentary from Dr. Harry Baum)

Education vs. Training: Is there a difference?

Training is defined as organized activity aimed at imparting information and/or instructions to improve the recipient's performance or to help him or her attain a required level of knowledge or skill. This usually occurs just one time and then is repeated as needed.

Education is the gaining of knowledge acquired by an individual after being instructed on a particular subject that provides an understanding of that subject. Education requires instruction of some sort from an individual. Education requires continuous follow-up until the process or subject is mastered.

BE SURE TO USE THE EDUCATIONAL PROCESS WHENEVER YOU CAN. IT IS THE ONLY WAY TO BREAK BAD HABITS AND TO AVOID RETURNING TO THEM.

(Contributed by Dr. Harry Baum)

NOTES:

_____
_____
_____
_____
_____
_____
_____
_____
_____
_____
_____
_____
_____
_____
_____
_____
_____
_____
_____
_____
_____
_____
_____
_____

Harry G. Baum, Ed.D

Made in the USA
Lexington, KY
11 November 2014